Calorie deficit cookbook

Unleash your weight-loss program with a high protein, guilt free and easy meal recipes to stay healthy

Bryan K. Keller

Copyright Page:

© [2024] [Bryan K. Keller]

ISBN:

Disclaimer: The information provided in this book is for educational and informational purposes only. The author and publisher are not liable for any losses or damages that may occur as a result of following the information presented in this book. Readers should consult with a qualified professional before making any significant changes to their lifestyle, health, or other aspects of their lives based on the content of this book.

Table of Contents

Chapter 1

Introduction

Understanding the calorie deficit concept

Welcome to your quest to become healthier and happy! In today's society, when many people prioritize wellbeing, knowing the calorie deficit idea is essential for accomplishing long-term weight reduction and health objectives.

At its foundation, the calorie deficit notion is based on an extremely straightforward yet encompassing approach: to shed weight, you must ingest a lower calorie content than your body puts out. In simple terms, it's centered on causing a deficit of energy by burning far more calories compared to your intake. Though this may appear simple, the complexities of successfully applying a calorie deficit plan are where the actual magic lies. In this in-depth guidance, we'll look at the rationale underlying the calorie deficit, its mechanism of operation, and the reason why it's such an important part of any effective weight reduction plan. We'll dispel common beliefs and misunderstandings, giving you the expertise and resources you require to explore the world of dietary habits with optimism.

However, calorie deficit is more than simply restriction and starvation; it is also about adopting decisions that feed your body while enabling you to eat the things you want. All through this trip, you'll find tasty and nutritious dishes designed to help you achieve your calorie deficit objectives, demonstrating that wholesome dining can be both pleasant and gratifying.

Perhaps you're just starting out on your weight reduction transition or are interested in optimizing your strategy; this book will help you succeed. So strap on and prepare to start on a transformational adventure to a healthier, happier self. With effort, persistence, and a solid knowledge of the calorie reduction principle, you may achieve the physique and lifestyles you've always desired.

In the following pages, we'll deconstruct the calorie reduction concept and break down the information into practical suggestions that you can apply into your everyday routine. From meal planning to social settings, we'll cover it everything, to make sure you have the understanding and skills you need to succeed on your weight reduction journey.

However, although the calorie deficit notion is an effective tool for weight reduction, it is only one component of the picture. A well-rounded strategy which involves regular physical exercise, appropriate water intake, and mindful eating is critical for long-term success.

Throughout this book, we'll provide you concrete suggestions, expert guidance, and tasty recipes to help you achieve your calorie deficit objectives. Whether you want a robust breakfast that will begin your day off well or a filling meal that finishes it on an optimistic note, we have you covered.

So, are you prepared to take the initial step toward a better, happier self? Let us get in and explore the transformational potential of the calorie reduction idea together. Your road toward a better lifestyle begins today.

The significance of Appropriate Nutrition for losing weight

Weight reduction is more than simply cutting calories; it's also about fueling the human body with the correct nutrients to promote good health as a whole. Here's a thorough look at how balanced diet might help you lose weight:

Maintaining Energy Levels

Taking a balanced meal, your body obtains a consistent amount of energy during the day. Having a combination of complex carbs, protein, and nutritious fats may help you prevent energy dips and maintain appropriate energy levels, which are essential for remaining energetic and shedding pounds.

Optimal Metabolism: Nourishing your organs with the necessary nutrition promotes a healthy metabolism. When you consume a well-balanced diet, your metabolism runs smoothly, helping you lose calories more quickly. This can help you avoid peaks in your weight reduction journey and encourage consistent, long-term improvement.

Muscle Maintenance: Maintaining lean muscle mass is critical while attempting to reduce weight. A well-balanced diet rich in protein promotes muscle development and repair, minimizing muscle loss during calorie restriction. Retaining muscle mass is beneficial to general endurance, metabolism, and the composition of the body.

Nutrient Absorption: A wide range of minerals, vitamins, and additional nutrients are required for normal body function. Eating a variety of nutrient-dense meals supports the way your body absorbs and uses these critical elements properly. This not only aids in weight reduction, but also improves general health and vigor.

Appetite Control: A well-balanced diet is important for controlling hunger and appetite. items packed in protein, fiber, and beneficial fats help you feel full and satisfied, lowering your chances of overeating or nibbling on high-calorie, low-nutrient items. This can lead to a decrease in overall calorie consumption, which can help with weight loss.

Improved Digestive Health: Consuming veggies, fruit, and whole-grain products, along with other fiber-rich diets promotes digestive wellness and regularity. A well-functioning digestive system helps all waste to be properly cleared from the body, resulting in less bloating and a flatter stomach. Furthermore, a healthy gut flora has been related to improved weight control and metabolism.

Balanced Hormones: Nutrition has an important influence in hormone control, which can affect hunger, metabolism, and the accumulation of fat. A well-rounded diet promotes hormonal equilibrium, which supports the normal function of hormones associated with weight management which include insulin, leptin levels and ghrelin.

Lifestyle Sustainability: Eating a well-balanced diet with a range of foods helps make sure your dietary needs are satisfied while providing opportunities for pleasure and adaptability. Sustainable lifestyle modifications are more likely to result in sustained weight loss achievement than limiting calories or excessive eating habits.

Finally, balanced diet is critical for weight reduction since it improves general health, energy levels, muscle mass preservation, hunger regulation, digestive health, hormone balance, and the development of sustainable lifestyle habits. Prioritizing nutrient-dense meals and keeping a well-rounded diet will help you lose weight as well as fueling your body for over a long period health and energy.

How to Use This Cookbook Effectively

Set Specific Goals: Before digging into those recipes, spend a moment to set your personal weight reduction objectives. Decide your desired weight loss, goal timeline, and any dietary preferences or limits. Having specific goals will allow you to personalize the way you prepare meals as well as make the most of the recipes available.

Plan Your Meals: Employ the recipes contained in this book as a starting point for your meal execution. Consider the numerous advantages of the mealtime and snack choices for creating balanced and fulfilling meals every week. Consider bulk cooking or meal preparing on weekend to save valuable time and ensuring you have healthy alternatives on hand.

Track Your Calories: Because the cookbook is based on the calorie deficit idea, you must track how many calories you consume to verify you are meeting your weight reduction objectives. Use a food journal or a calorie monitoring software to keep track of your daily calorie intake and change portion sizes whenever necessary to sustain a calorie deficit.

Mix & Match Recipes: Do not be scared to combine recipes to fit your tastes and dietary requirements. Feel free to substitute items, modify portion proportions, or blend recipes to create unique meals that reflect your taste interests and calorie objectives. Get imaginative and try new taste combos to make your meals interesting and rewarding.

Maintain Consistency: Consistency is essential for long-term weight reduction success. Commit to incorporate dishes from this cook book into your regular routine, and prioritize healthy eating habits.

Strive to adhere to the deficit-calorie plan regularly, but keep in mind to give yourself some leeway and enjoyment by indulging in snacks or eating out in moderation.

Listen to your body. Keep an eye to the way your body reacts to the foods you're eating. Consider how certain meals make you feel invigorated and satiated, whereas others might leave you feeling lethargic or bloated. Use this input to make informed diet decisions and change your food plan accordingly to maximize your weight reduction results.

Stay Motivated: Celebrating your accomplishments along the road can help you remain inspired and intent on your weight reduction objectives. Celebrate little triumphs, such as reaching new goals or regularly adhering to your dietary regimen, and appreciate yourself using non-food prizes to keep you motivated and inspired along the way.

By adopting these guidelines and using the recipes and tactics outlined in this cooking book, you will be able to properly exploit the effectiveness of the calorie shortage idea to reach your weight reduction objectives and begin on a road to better health and wellness.

Chapter 2
Embracing the Calorie Deficit Lifestyle

What is Calorie Deficit, and how does it work

Being acquainted with the notion of a shortage of calories is critical for successful weight reduction. A calorie shortage happens when you eat a lesser number of calories compared to what your body requires to maintain its present weight. Let's go into the specifics of what a deficit in calories is and the way it works.

Defining a Calorie Deficit

A calorie shortfall is the difference between the calories you ingest from meals and beverages and the calories you expend via metabolism and physical exercise. It is crucial to understand that not all of the calories have been made equal. While the number of calories counts for weight reduction, the nutritional content of those calories is as important for general health and well-being.

How It Works

To shed weight, your body must be in a negative energy balance, meaning it burns more calories than it takes in. This causes your body to use its energy resources (mainly fat) to compensate for the shortage, resulting in weight reduction over time.

Your body needs a specific amount of calorie intake each day for keeping its present weight, which is known as Total Daily Energetic Expenses (TDEE). This comprises calories required for fundamental body activities (base metabolic rate), physical exercise, and the thermal effect of meals.

By generating a shortage of calories, you compel the human body to use energy stored reserves (which can include body fat) to fulfill its energy requirements, which results in weight reduction.

For instance, if the total daily energy expenditure (TDEE) is 3,000 calories each day whereas you only eat 2,500 calories, you're producing a 500-calorie deficit every day. Over time, this deficiency causes an overall reduction of body weight.

Determining Your Calorie Deficit

The very first step in determining your calorie deficit is to calculate your use (a TDEE). This may be achieved by utilizing online calculators or formulae that take into consideration variables which include age, sex, height, weight, and activity level.

Once you've calculated your total daily energy expenditure, you may create a nutritional deficit by eating a smaller amount of calories than your The total daily energy expenditure. A frequent strategy is to maintain a small deficit in calories of 500 to 750 per day, which usually results in a slow and consistent pace of weight reduction.

It's vital to realize that generating an excessive calorie deficit might result in muscle loss, vitamin shortages, metabolic slowness, and other negative consequences. As a result, it's typically suggested to strive for a minor shortfall that allows for consistent improvement while still supplying your system with the nutrition and energy it requires to function properly.

Monitoring Progress

Monitoring your progress on a frequent basis is critical to ensuring that you're efficiently producing a deficit in calories and moving toward your weight reduction objectives. This may be accomplished by tracking modifications to how much you weigh, measurements, and clothing fit.

Furthermore, tracking your food consumption using a food journal or calories tracking software will assist you remain accountable and discover areas in which you might have to make changes to keep up your calorie deficit.

It's crucial to realize that weight reduction progress isn't always linear, and there may be swings owing to things including water retention, hormonal shifts, and dietary changes. To effectively track your development, focus on trends over time rather than short-term variations.

Balanced Nutrition and Exercise

While having a shortage of calories is critical for weight reduction, it is also crucial to prioritize balanced diet and frequent physical exercise. A diet high in nutrient-dense foods, which includes fruits, vegetables, lean meats, whole-grain products, and healthy fats, supplies your body with the resources it requires to maintain good health and wellness.

Regular exercise not only helps you burn more calories, but it also boosts cardiovascular health, muscle strength, mood improvement, and general fitness. To get the most out of your reduced-calorie efforts, combine aerobic, strength, and flexibility activities.

It's critical to choose things you like and make physical exercise a permanent part of your life. Keep in mind that exercise does not need to be strenuous or lengthy to be beneficial. Even little modifications, for instance using staircases rather than the escalator or opting for a quick walk during lunchtime, can help you lose calories and improve your overall health.

Knowing how to calculate your calorie deficit, tracking your accomplishments, and including balanced dietary and physical activity into your routine will allow you to effectively use the calorie shortage concept to accomplish your weight loss goals while also improving your general well-being and health.

Sustainability and Adaptation

Sustainability is essential when adopting a calorie restriction for weight reduction. Extreme deficits or too restricted diets may produce rapid results at first, but they are frequently difficult to sustain over time, perhaps leading to rebound weight gain.

It's critical to discover a deficit of calories that works for you, taking into account your lifestyle, tastes, and metabolic demands. Gradual, steady growth is more durable and leads to lasting achievement than abrupt, radical changes.

Furthermore, your body may adjust to a calorie shortage over time, limiting weight reduction efforts. This is referred to as metabolic adaptation, or the "hunger mode" myth. While metabolic adaptation occurs to some level, it is often less significant than previously thought and may be minimized by modifying your calorie intake on a regular basis and integrating refeeding days.

Potential Challenges and Factors to consider

Developing and sustaining a shortage of calories may be difficult for certain people, particularly those with previous instances of an eating disorder or metabolic disorders. It is critical to look at shedding pounds with a healthy and sustained perspective, obtaining assistance from healthcare experts or registered dietitians as needed.

The effects of stress, disturbed sleep, hormones, and medical issues can all affect how your body reacts to a calorie shortage. Take note to how these elements influence your weight reduction journey and make changes as needed to improve your overall health.

It is also vital to recognize that calorie consumption and expenditure are not the only factors influencing weight reduction. Genetic variables, environmental effects, and psychological components which include stress, emotions, and behaviors all have a substantial impact on weight control results.

Finally, knowing the calorie deficit principle is critical for successful weight reduction. You may lose weight while improving your general wellness and health by generating a persistent deficit in calories through a mix of balanced nutrition, frequent physical exercise, and lifestyle changes.

Understand that losing weight is a journey, and the outcomes may differ from individual to individual. Be patient, consistent, and focused on making modest, long-term improvements that promote your health and happiness. With effort, perseverance, and a thorough knowledge of the deficit of calories idea, you may achieve successful outcomes on your weight reduction quest.

Benefits of Following a Calorie Deficit Diet

Maintaining a lower-calorie diet has various advantages beyond weight reduction. Here's a comprehensive peek at few of the major benefits:

Weight Loss: A calorie shortage diet is mostly beneficial for weight reduction. By continually ingesting fewer calories than the body spends, you developed a nutritional imbalance that causes your body to break down stored body fat for fuel, resulting in weight loss over time.

Improved Body Composition: A lower-calorie diet can enhance body composition by lowering body fat percentage and retaining lean muscle mass. This can lead to a healthier and defined figure.

Improved Metabolic Health: A low-calorie diet can enhance a variety of metabolic health indices, including blood sugar, insulin sensitivity, and cholesterol. A calorie deficit diet, which promotes weight loss and reduces excess fat formation, can minimize the risk of maladies related to obesity including type 2 diabetes and coronary heart disease.

Increased Energy Levels: Unlike common perception, a low-calorie diet does not always result in lower energy levels. In fact, many individuals report feeling more energized and alert after eating a balanced, nutrient-dense meal that supports their weight reduction objectives. Taking nutritious foods that give continuous energy can help you prevent energy drops and maintain peak level of energy throughout the day.

Enhanced mood and mental wellness: There is emerging evidence that dietary habits, especially calorie consumption, might influence mental well-being and mood. A calorie-deficit diet that focuses on full, nutrient-dense foods can improve mood, reduce stress, and boost cognitive performance. Furthermore, meeting weight loss objectives can enhance self-esteem and confidence, hence boosting mental health.

Improved Sleep Quality: Weight loss with a calorie-deficit diet has been related to better sleep duration and quality. Excessive body weight and poor food habits can both contribute to sleep disorders which include sleeping apnea and insomnia. A low-calorie diet can help improve sleep hygiene and quality by encouraging weight reduction and the adoption of healthy lifestyle practices.

Long-term Health Benefits: Aside from the immediate benefits of shedding weight, a low-calorie diet can provide a lifetime of health advantages that go far beyond physical appearance. Keeping an appropriate weight and following good living practices can lower your chance of developing chronic diseases including type 2 diabetes, coronary heart disease, some malignancies, and even Alzheimer's illness.

In general, a low-calorie diet can enhance weight, body structure, metabolic health, energy, state of mind, quality of sleep, and long-term health results. However, it is critical to work toward shedding pounds in a healthy and sustainable manner, emphasizing nutrient-dense diets, frequent physical exercise, and general well-being.

Tips for Creating a Sustainable Calorie Deficit Plan

Developing a viable decreased-calorie strategy is essential for lasting weight reduction success without jeopardizing your wellness or a healthy lifestyle. Listed below are some organized and straightforward guidelines to help you create a sustained calorie deficit plan:

Calculate Your Caloric Needs

Use an internet calculator or visit a healthcare expert to figure out your own Total Day Energy Expense (TDEE). This will offer you with an initial estimate of the number of calories required to keep up your current weight.

Set realistic goals.

Strive for a calorie shortage of 500 to 750 per day, which usually leads to a weight reduction of between one and two pounds every week. Setting reasonable and attainable objectives can help you maintain motivation and avoid emotions of deprivation or discontent.

Monitor your food intake

Create a food journal or use a calorie monitoring app to measure your daily calorie consumption. When you record food, snacks, and beverages, be honest and accurate. Pay close attention to portion proportions and ingredient proportions to guarantee accuracy.

Focus on Nutrient-Dense Foods

Stock your plate with nutrient-dense meals including fruits and vegetables, lean meats, whole grain foods, and wholesome fats. These meals are not only low in calories, but they also include important minerals, antioxidants, and vitamins that promote general health and well-being.

Practice Portion Regulation

Be cautious of size of portions to steer clear of overeating, especially while eating healthful meals.

Use small plates, bowls, and cutlery to keep portion sizes under control, and stay away from inconsiderate consumption by focusing close consideration to satiety and fullness signs.

Prioritize protein and fiber: Incorporate lean proteins and fiber-rich foods in the form of snacks and meals to boost feelings of contentment and pleasure. Protein-rich meals like chicken, fish, vegetarian tofu, Greek yoghurt and beans will help you maintain lean muscle mass while losing weight

Minimize added sugars and packaged foods: Reduce your use of sugary beverages, candies, processed snacks, as well as high-calorie comfort meals. These meals are frequently poor in nutrition and rich in unneeded calories, making it simple to surpass your calorie limit without feeling full.

Remain hydrated: Consume lots of water through the day to keep hydrated and promote good health. Thirst can be misunderstood for hunger, resulting in needless munching or eating excessively. Try to drink 8-10 glasses of water every day, even more if you are more active or stay in a hot environment.

Incorporate physical activity: While nutrition plays an important part in shedding pounds, frequent workouts can boost calorie burn and support overall health. Consider activities you love, which might include biking, walking, diving, or dancing, and commit to a minimum of 150 minutes of moderately intense exercise every week.

Listen to your body: Keep an eye to the way your body reacts to your calorie-deficit strategy. If you find yourself too hungry, tired, or deprived, it might be an indication that the deficit in calories is too extreme. Be adaptable and change your approach as needed to strike a balance that's suitable for you.

Plan beforehand and prepare meals. Schedule your snacks and meals ahead of time to make sure that you always have nutritional alternatives on hand.

Combining recipes on weekend or meal planning for the coming week ahead may save time and make a nutritious diet more easy, lowering the temptation to go for harmful quick foods or processed snacks.

Include treats in moderation: Letting yourself the odd treat or indulgence might help you avoid feeling of deprivation and stick to your low-calorie diet strategy. To prevent derailing your progress, consume these indulgences in moderation and fit them into your total calorie budget.

Practice Mindful Eating: Calm down and focus on your dietary routine by learning mindful eating. Take time to enjoy each meal, chew fully, and pay attention to your own body's feelings of fullness and hunger signals. To prevent overeating, avoid distractions like devices and multitasking while eating.

Seek support and accountability: Spend time with a supporting circle of relatives, close companions, and online groups that support and inspire you on your weight reduction journey. Consider hiring a licensed nutritionist, personal fitness instructor, or weight reduction coach to provide further direction and accountability.

Monitor progress and modify as needed: Regularly assess your progress toward your weight reduction objectives and change your calorie deficit strategy as needed. If you reach a plateau or encounter difficulties, evaluate your food habits, exercise levels, and general lifestyle to discover areas for improvement.

Emphasis on Non-Scale Victories: While weight reduction is a typical aim of calorie deficit diets, it's also important to recognize non-scale wins along the road. Improved energy levels, physical wellness, mood, quality of sleep, and overall well-being will serve as markers of your improvement and achievement.

Be patient and persistent: Remember that lasting weight reduction requires time and perseverance. It is common to face challenges and disappointments along your journey, but consistencies as well as persistence are essential. Maintain focus on your long-term objectives and remind yourself that gradual and steady development is far more probable to lead to permanent outcomes.

Celebrate Your Successes: Take time to recognize your accomplishments and developments, no matter how minor. Recognize your successes and celebrate yourself with non-food incentives that correspond with your beliefs and interests, whether it's completing a mini-goal, adhering to your plan for a set length of time, or conquering a hurdle.

By adding these recommendations into your low-calorie diet plan, you can develop a long-term weight reduction strategy that supports your objectives while also boosting general health and well-being. Remember that each path is unique, so figure out which method works most effectively for you and enjoy the adventure of becoming the most fit and healthy version of yourself.

Chapter 3
Energizing Breakfasts

Nutrient-Dense Morning Meals to Jumpstart Your Day

Protein-Rich Breakfast Bowl

Ingredients: Quinoa with scrambled eggs or vegan tofu, lettuce, cherry tomatoes, avocados slices, and feta cheese.

Instructions: Prepare the quinoa in accordance to package directions. In a separate skillet, combine eggs or tofu, lettuce, and cherry tomatoes. Serve the quinoa with the egg and tofu combination, avocados slices, and a sprinkling of feta cheese.

Greek Yogurt Parfait

Ingredients: Greek yogurt, a blend of berries (strawberries, blueberry preserves, and raspberry), almonds or walnuts as well, chia seeds, and optional honey or maple syrup drizzle.

Instructions: In a glass or dish, combine Greek yogurt, mixed berries, almonds, and chia seeds. If you want to add more sweetness, drizzle with maple syrup or honey.

Vegetable Omelette on Whole Grain Toast
Ingredients: Eggs, red bell peppers, onion slices, spinach, mushrooms, whole wheat bread, and a garnish of salsa or avocados.

Instructions: To prepare, whisk the eggs and throw them into a hot skillet. Include diced red bell peppers, onions, lettuce, and mushrooms. Cook till the eggs have set, then fold them in half. Serve with whole grain bread with salsa or avocado.

Whole Grain Pancakes and Nut Butter and Bananas
Ingredients: whole grain pancakes blend (or homemade batters), almonds or peanut butter, a sliced banana, and cinnamon.

Instructions: Make pancakes according to the package guidelines or your preferred recipe. Spread the nut cream on over of the pancake and decorate with sliced banana. Decorate with cinnamon for extra taste.

Smoothie bowl

Ingredients: Mixing frozen berries, bananas, greens or kale, Greek or plant-based food yogurt, almond milk, or water from coconuts, and top like granola, chopped fruit, nuts, and seed.

Instructions: Blend together frozen berries, banana, greens or kale, yogurt, and the almond milk or water from coconuts until smooth. Pour into a bowl and garnish with granola, chopped fruit, nut, and seed for extra flavor and nutrition.

Avocado toast and poached eggs: The ingredients include whole grain bread, ripened avocado, poached eggs, cherry tomatoes, black pepper, and sea salt.

Instructions: Preheat whole grain loaf and spread mashed mature avocado on top. Add a poached egg on over the avocados and decorate with sliced cherry tomatoes. Add black pepper & sea salt as desired.

These rich in nutrients morning meals are high in vitamins, minerals, fiber, and protein, which will help you stay energized throughout the day. Explore with various ingredient and taste combinations to see which one works best for you, and have a delightful start to the day!

Quick and Easy Breakfast Recipes for Busy Mornings

Overnight oat

Ingredients: Rolled oatmeal, milk (dairy products or plant-based food), Greek yogurt, beeswax or maple syrup, and optional fruit, nuts, and seed.

Instruction: To make the recipe, mix the oats, yogurt, milk and the desired sweetener in a dish or jar. Stir thoroughly, cover, and chill overnight. Stir the oats in the morning and top with your preferred toppings before eating.

Whole grain toast and nut butter

Ingredients include whole- grain bread, nut butter (almond, pcanuts, or cashew), and fruit cut into pieces (bananas, berries, or apple slices).

Instructions: Toast the whole grain bread till golden brown. Spread nut butter over top and garnish with sliced fruit for more taste and nutrition. Serve it alongside a glass of milk and a slice of stringy cheese for extra protein.

Greek yogurt with fruit parfait

Greek yogurt, various berries (including strawberries, blueberries, and raspberry), granola, and a sprinkle of honey or maple syrup as desired (optional). In a container or dish, combine Greek yogurt, mixed berries, and granola. Repeat layers as desired, and then top with a small amount of honey and maple syrup for taste. Enjoy now or take it with you!

Quick Breakfast Burritos

Ingredients: a whole-grain tortilla, egg scrambles, black beans, cubed avocados, salsa, and crumbled cheese (optional).

Instructions: Warm up your tortillas in the skillet or microwave. Optional toppings include egg scramble, black beans, sliced avocados salsa, and shredded cheese. Roll up a burrito and eat as is, or wrap it in wrap for an easily carried breakfast

Smoothie on the Go: Ingredients: Frozen fruit (such berries or tropical fruits), bananas, greens or kale, powdered protein or greek yoghurt, and almond milk or water from coconuts.

Instructions: Blend together frozen fruit, banana, greens, Greek yogurt or protein powder, and almond milk or coconut water. Blend until smooth, adding additional liquid if required. Pour into a travel cup or Mason jar for an easy breakfast on-the-go.

Microwave Egg Mug

Ingredients: Eggs, milk (optional), chopped veggies (include peppers, onion slices, and greens), shredded cheese, and spices.

Instructions: In a microwave-safe cup, combine the eggs, milk, chopped veggies, shredded cheese, and spices. Microwaves at a high temperature for one to two minutes, turning halfway through, until the eggs have set. Serve hot along with whole grain toasts or English muffins.

The aforementioned simple and fast breakfast dishes are ideal for those hectic mornings when you desire a nutritious meal quickly. With minimum meal planning and cooking duration, you may have a tasty and filling breakfast to power your day. Feel free to add your preferred components and flavors to these recipes for more variation and enjoyment!

Incorporating Protein and Fiber for Long-Lasting Energy

Start with a Balanced Breakfast

Start off your day with a meal for breakfast that includes proteins and fiber-rich foods. Options include Greek yogurt with a variety of fruits and granola, as well as whole grain toast with avocados and poached eggs.

Snack smartly

Choose protein and fiber-rich snacks to keep you full in between meals. For instance, slices of apples with almond cream, carrots with hummus, and an insignificant scoop with nuts and seeds.

Load up on veggies

Add lots of veggies to your meals to increase your fiber intake. Fill half of the plate with non-starchy veggies including leafy greens, broccoli, among others, peppers, and cauliflower. Add grilled chicken, tofu-based or legumes for protein.

Choose whole grains

Choose whole grains like quinoa, brown rice, and oatmeal, as well as whole wheat bread, spaghetti, and crackers. These grains are high in fiber and offer a consistent source of energy. For a well-balanced dinner, serve alongside lean protein sources such as grilled fish or lentils.

Include protein in each meal

Include a protein source in each meal to help with muscle regeneration and to keep you satiated. Lean meats, seafood, eggs, poultry, dairy goods, tofu, tempeh, lentils, and nuts are all excellent protein sources.

Snack on fiber-rich fruits

Include fiber-rich fruits like berries, pears, apples, citrus fruits, and kiwi in your meals and snacks. The fruits mentioned above are not only tasty, but also provide an excellent amount of vitamins and minerals or antioxidant.

Snack on fibre-rich nuts and seeds

To increase your protein and fiber consumption, munch on just a few pieces of nuts and seeds. Almonds are walnuts, pistachio chia seeds, hemp seeds, and flax seeds are all wonderful choices for a delicious crunch and a variety of nutrients

Stay Hydrated

Stay hydrated by drinking enough of water through the day to promote digestion and maintain energy levels. Foods high in fiber absorb water, so staying hydrated is vital to avoiding constipation and maintaining general health.

Balance your Plate

Balance your plate with protein, fiber-rich carbs, healthy fats, and veggies. This balance will assist to maintain blood sugar levels, minimize energy breaks down, and keep you satiated for longer.

By adopting these guidelines into your everyday dietary routine, you can guarantee that your body receives the nutrients it requires for long-term vitality and good health. Remember to eat nutritious, minimally processed meals and heed to your body's signals for feeling of fullness and hunger cues to improve your overall health.

Chapter 4
Nourishing Lunches

Healthy and Filling Lunch Ideas to Keep You Satisfied

Grilled Chicken Salad

Ingredients: Grilled chicken breast, avocado slices, bell peppers, cucumbers, cherry tomatoes, and mixed greens with a balsamic vinaigrette.

Instructions: Combine chopped bell peppers, cherry tomatoes, cucumber slices, mixed greens, and avocado slices. Add a cooked chicken breast on top and garnish it with balsamic vinaigrette.

Quinoa & Black Bean Bowl

Ingredients: boiled quinoa, black beans, corn kernels, sliced avocado for garnish, salsa, and lime wedges; vegetables include sautéed with bell peppers and onions.

Instructions: Mix chopped avocado, black beans, sautéed onions and bell peppers, and corn kernels with cooked quinoa. Garnish with fresh lime juice and salsa.

Wrap with turkey and hummus

Ingredients: Shredded carrots, cucumber slices, hummus, sliced turkey breast, spinach as well as mixed greens, and whole wheat wrap.

Instruction

Take a whole wheat-based wrap, spread some hummus on it, then top with slices of cucumber, shredded carrots, spinach as well as mixed greens, and turkey breast. Cut in half after firmly rolling up.

Peppers Stuffed with Quinoa and Salmon

Ingredients

Flaked cooked salmon, cooked quinoa, diced tomatoes, chopped spinach, and grated mozzarella cheese are the ingredients.

Instructions: Slice the bell peppers in half and take out the seeds. Add cooked quinoa, flaked salmon, diced tomatoes, chopped spinach, and grated mozzarella cheese to the inside of the bowl. Melt cheese and soften peppers by baking.

Mediterranean Salad with Chickpeas

Ingredients: Include chopped parsley, crumbled feta cheese, tomatoes with cherries, red onion, sliced cucumbers, shredded parsley, and a dressing made of lemon and olive oil.

Instructions

Add chopped parsley, crumbled feta cheese, sliced red onion, chopped cucumbers, split cherry tomatoes, and Kalamata olives to the chickpea mixture. Dress with a lemon-olive oiled mixture and toss.

Stir-fried vegetables with tofu

Ingredients include sesame oil, ginger, garlic, soy sauce, bell peppers, cauliflower, snapping peas, and carrot stir-fried in a mixture of veggies. The tofu is firm.

Instructions

In a pan, sauté cubed firm tofu, mixed stir-fry veggies, garlic, and ginger until the vegetables are crisp-tender. Add some soy sauce and sesame oil for seasoning.

Roasted vegetables and pesto paired with whole grain pasta

Ingredients: Grated Parmesan cheese, roasted veggies (such as tomatoes with cherry flavor, the zucchini, red bell peppers, and red onion), whole grain pasta, and handmade or store-bought pesto sauce.

Instructions

Follow the cooking directions on the package for whole grain pasta. Add roasted veggies and toss with pesto sauce. Sprinkle grated Parmesan cheese over top and serve.

Avocado Stuffed with Tuna Salad:

Ingredients: Ripe avocados, Greek yogurt, sliced celery, diced red onions, lemon juice, and salt & pepper.

Instructions

Combine Greek yogurt, chopped celery, red onion, lime juice salt, and peppers with the canned tuna. Pit ripe avocados by cutting them in half. Top each half of an avocado with a portion of tuna salad.

Sweet potato and black bean quesadillas

Ingredients: Black beans, mashed sweet potatoes, salsa, shredded cheese, chopped jalapeños (optional), whole wheat tortillas.

Instructions: Take a complete wheat tortilla and spread one side with mashed sweet potatoes. Add chopped jalapeños, shredded cheese, and black beans on top, if you want. In a pan, fold the flour tortilla in halves and cook till golden and crisp on both sides. Present alongside salsa.

Mason jars Salad

Ingredients: Toss to combine the preferred salad mixture in a mason jar; pour dressing in the bottom and top with plenty

Ingredients: Include grains or beans, followed by veggies, proteins, and, for garnish, greens. When it's time to dine, stir the jar to release the dressing and dig in!

Packed with nutrients, these satisfying lunch ideas will keep you full and energized all day long. For fun and diversity, feel free to alter the recipes to include your preferred flavors and ingredients!

Portable Lunch Options for Work or School
Wrap It Up
Turkey along with Cheese Wrap: Place cheese, lettuce, tomato, and sliced turkey breast within a whole wheat wrap. To make it easier to travel, split it in half and roll it securely.

Veggie Hummus Wrap: Spread a whole wheat wrapper with hummus, then top with cucumber, bell pepper, carrot, and spinach slices. Roll it up and cover it with parchment paper or foil.

Bento Box Treasures:

Bento Box Packed with Protein: Arrange cucumber slices, cherry tomatoes, hard-boiled eggs, grilled chicken breast slices, and whole wheat crackers into the partitions of a bento box.

Bento Box with a Mediterranean Theme: Stuff sections with feta cheese cubes, tomatoes with cherries, cucumbers slices, olives, and hummus made from whole wheat pita bread.

Salad Jars:

Mason jar Salad: Stack your preferred salad mixture in a mason jar, starting with the dressing and working your way up to hearty elements like grains or beans, then veggies, proteins, and greens. When it's time to dine, shake the container to spread the dressing.

Quinoa Salad Jar: Put cooked quinoa, diced veggies, chick peas feta cheese, and various greens in a mason jar. Dressing should be packed separately and added just when willing to eat.

Portable protein boxes

Make your own protein box by packing a segmented container with eggs that have been hard-boiled, cheese cubes, and sliced deli meat, almonds or trails mix, and apples or grape.

Nut Cream and Fruit Box: Sprinkle small amounts of nut butter over whole grain cracker or rice cakes and mix with sliced apples.

Soup in an insulated container

Make your preferred soups or chili and put it in an insulated container to retain it hot until noon. For a substantial supper, serve with whole wheat crackers or crusty toast.

Cold Soups Alternative: A gazpacho or chill cucumber soup may be packaged in an insulated container for a cool lunch on hot days.

DIY Snack Boxes
Mix and combine portable snacks like cheese sticks, whole wheat crackers, freshly picked fruit, baby carrots, humus containers, yogurt boxes, and granola bars. Put these in a lunch container or thermo bag for convenient snacking during the day.

Repurpose leftovers to a portable lunch. Place grilled chicken alongside roasted veggies, tossed tofu alongside brown rice, or spaghetti salad with mixed vegetables in a microwave-safe dish.

These easy and planned portable lunches are ideal for bringing to the workplace or school. With a little forethought and planning, you can have a nutritious and filling dinner on the move!

Tips for Balancing Macronutrients in Lunchtime Meals

Add Lean Protein

For lunch, include a lean protein source, such as fish, beans, lentils, tempeh, tofu, or grilled chicken breast. Aim for a serving size that is comparable to your palm.

Insert Nutritious Carbohydrates

Incorporate complex carbs to give you energy that lasts all day. Select whole grains like quinoa, brown rice, sweet potatoes, chickpeas, black beans, and whole-grain bread or pasta.

Remember the Good Fats

Add some heart-healthy fats to your packed lunch to help with nutrition absorption and fullness. Drizzle salads or roasted veggies with olive oil, add sliced avocado, almonds, and seeds.

Eat a Lot of Vegetables

Non-starchy vegetables like greens, spinach, bell peppers, the cucumber, tomato products, broccoli, or carrots should make up at least part of your lunch plate. Vegetables are rich in vitamins, minerals, and fiber yet low in calories.

Balanced portions

By picturing your plate, try to balance the amounts of your macronutrients by filling half of it with fruits and vegetables, a quarter of the with proteins, and one-quarter with carbs. Adapt portion sizes to your level of exercise and unique energy requirements.

Select Whole Foods

Whenever possible, choose whole, minimally processed meals. Select whole grains instead of refined ones, and go for fresh produce wherever possible rather than processed or canned goods.

Maintain Hydration

To keep hydrated all day, remember to have water with your meal. Try to drink 8–10 glasses of water or more if you work out or are in a hot climate each day.

Make a Plan

To guarantee that your lunches are wholesome and well-balanced, prepare them in advance. Prepare items in advance to make lunch assembly quick and simple. Examples of this include cutting vegetables and boiling grains and meats.

Pay Attention to Your Body

Consider how different foods affect your mood and modify your midday diet accordingly. Observe how well-balanced meals affect your satiety, energy, and general health.

Try Different Textures and Flavors

Try experimenting with new taste, feel, and cuisines to keep your meals interesting. To keep your meals tasty and fulfilling, experiment with different culinary delights, spices, and cooking techniques.

You can quickly prepare nutritious midday meals that provide your body the nutrition it needs to flourish by adhering to these easy suggestions. In order to maintain your health and wellbeing, always pay attention to your body's signals of hunger and fullness and modify as necessary.

Chapter 5
Satisfying Dinners

Wholesome Dinner Recipes for Every Palate

Roasted vegetables with grilled chicken with herbs and spices:

Ingredients:

a. Four skinless, boneless chicken breasts are the ingredients:

b. Two tsp olive oil

c. One lemon's juice

d. Two minced garlic cloves

e. A single tsp of dried thyme

f. One tsp of dehydrated rosemary

g. To taste, add salt and pepper.

h. Chopped bell peppers, a zucchini, the carrots, and red onions, among other veggies.

Instructions

The mixture of olive oil, lime juice, chopped garlic, and dried thyme leaves dried rosemary extract, salt, and pepper should all be combined in a small bowl.

Pour the marinade on the chicken breasts and place them in a plastic bag that can be sealed. After sealing the bag, let it marinade for at least half an hour in the fridge.

Grill at a medium-high temperature. Take the chicken out of the marinade and throw away any extra marinade.

Chicken should be cooked thoroughly and no longer pinkish in the center after 6 to 8 minutes on each side of the grill.

In the meantime, combine chopped veggies with salt, pepper, and olive oil. Arrange them evenly on a sheet of parchment paper and bake at 400 degrees Fahrenheit (200 degrees Celsius) for 20 to 25 minutes at a time, or until they become soft and have a hint of caramelization.

For a tasty and nutritious meal, pair grilled lemon herbs chicken with roasted veggies supper.

Bell peppers stuffed with quinoa

Ingredients

a. Four big bell peppers, seeded and halved

b. One cup of washed quinoa

c. Two cups water or vegetable broth

d. One tablespoon of olive oil

e. One chopped onion

f. Two minced garlic cloves

g. One can (15 ounces) of rinsed and drained black beans

h. One cup of fresh, frozen, or tinned corn kernels

i. One teaspoon of cumin powder

j. One tsp of chili powder

h. Add pepper and sea salt to taste. Add one cup of shredded cheese if desired.

Instructions

Turn the oven on to 375°F, or 190°C. Halve the bell peppers and place them in a baking tray.

Bring water or vegetable broth to a boil in a medium saucepan. After adding the quinoa, lower the heat to a simmer, cover, and let the quinoa cook for 15 to 20 minutes, until all of the liquid has been absorbed.

Heat the olive oil in a big skillet over medium heat. Cook for approximately five minutes, or until the diced onion and garlic minced are tender.

Add the cooked quinoa, which black beans, kernels of corn, chili powder, ground cumin, salt, and pepper, and stir. Cook for a further two to three minutes, or until well heated.

Fill bell pepper halves with quinoa mixture, gently pushing to compact.

Top the filled bell peppers with shredded cheese, if using.

Once the peppers are soft and the mixture is well cooked, bake the baking dish covered with foil for 25 to 30 minutes.

Serve the spicy bell peppers with quinoa filling, topped with chopped green onions or fresh cilantro, if preferred.

Easy One-Pot Vegetable and Lentil Curry

Ingredients

a. One tablespoon of olive oil

b. One chopped onion

c. Two minced garlic cloves

d. One spoonful of curry powder

e. One teaspoon of cumin powder

f. One tsp finely ground turmeric

g. 1 cup washed and drained dried lentils, either brown or green

h. Three cups of broth made from vegetables

i. One can, or fourteen ounces chopped tomatoes

j. Two cups of finely chopped veggies, such spinach, bell peppers, the cauliflower plant, and carrots

k. To taste, add salt and pepper.

l. Naan bread or cooked rice ready to be served

Instructions

Heat the olive oil in a big saucepan or Dutch oven over medium heat. Cook for approximately five minutes, or until the onion diced and minced garlic are tender.

Add the ground turmeric, cumin, and curry powder and stir. Cook for a further one to two minutes, or until aromatic.

To the saucepan, add chopped tomatoes, vegetable broth, and dry lentils. After bringing to a boil, lower heat to a simmer, cover, and cook for 20 to 25 minutes, until the lentils are soft.

Cook the chopped veggies for a further five to seven minutes, or until they are soft.

To taste, add salt and pepper for seasoning.

For a filling and substantial supper, serve hot one-pot lentils and vegetable stew over prepared rice or along with naan bread.

These healthy, straightforward meal dishes are simple to make and can be tailored to your preferred ingredients to fit any kind of palette. Savor a tasty and wholesome dinner that the entire family will appreciate!

One-Pot Meals for Easy Cleanup and Preparation

One-Pot Chicken and Vegetable Quinoa

Ingredients

a. One tablespoon of olive oil

b. One pound of skinless, boneless chicken breasts, sliced into small pieces

c. One little onion, chopped

d. Two minced garlic cloves

e. One cup of rinsed and drained quinoa

f. Two cups of chicken stock

g. 1 cup chopped tomatoes, either fresh or canned

h. One cup of finely diced veggies, such carrots, zucchini, and bell peppers

i. A single tsp of dried thyme

j. One tsp of dehydrated oregano

k. To taste, add salt and pepper.

l. Chopped fresh parsley (optional garnish)

Instructions

Take the pan off the burner as soon as the quinoa is fully cooked and nearly every drop of the liquid has been absorbed. If needed, adjust the seasoning by tasting it.

If preferred, top the hot one-pot chicken and veggie quinoa with freshly chopped parsley.

The chicken, quinoa, which and veggies in this dish are not only very nutritious and quick to make, but they are also a great source of protein and fiber. Plus, it simplifies cleanup after supper because there is just one pot to wash!

Strategies for Reducing Caloric Intake without Sacrificing Flavor

Several crucial tactics may be used to save calories without compromising flavor:

Concentrate on Whole Foods: Create a foundation for your meals by incorporating only lightly processed whole foods such fruits, vegetables, whole grains, lean meats, and healthy fats. When compared to refined foods, these foods are often higher in nutrients and fewer in calories.

Portion Control: Be mindful of serving sizes and try to load your plate with the right amounts of every food category. To assist in visually controlling portion sizes, use smaller bowls and plates.

Include Tasty Herbs and Spices: Try varying the herbs, spices, plus aromatics in your food to give it taste without increasing the calorie count. Spices like turmeric, paprika, and cumin, together with fresh herbs like mint, basil, and cilantro, can improve the flavor of your food.

Select Low-Calorie Cooking Techniques: Go for cooking techniques like grilling, baking, steaming, grilling, or broiling that call for the least amount of additional fat. With the help of these techniques, you may savor food's natural tastes without consuming extra calories from additional fats or oils.

Use Healthy Fats Caution: Although fats are necessary for taste and fullness, they are high in calories. Use healthy fats sparingly to enhance the flavor and richness of your meals, such as those found in nuts, seeds, avocados, olive oil, and avocado.

Boost Your Intake of Fiber: Include foods high in fiber in your meals, such as veggies, fruits, grains, legumes, and nuts. Fiber lowers the chance of overeating by increasing satiety and prolonging the sense of fullness.

Be Aware of Liquid Calories: Watch out for liquid calories from alcoholic drinks, sugar-filled beverages, and calorically dense coffee drinks. Instead, go for water, green tea, or sparkling liquid flavored with a little lime or lemon.

Plan and Cook Meals at Home: You can better manage the ingredients and portion amounts when you cook at home. Make a list of your meals and prepare healthy dishes in bulk so you may have them ready for the week.

Lean Protein Sources to Consider: Skinless chicken, fish, tofu, tempeh, lentils, and lower-fat dairy products are examples of lean protein sources. These choices offer protein and other necessary elements without adding too many calories.

Eat mindfully by taking your time, enjoying every meal, and focusing on the tastes, textures, and sensations you encounter. You may avoid eating too much and feel more pleased with lesser servings when you eat attentively.

You may lower your calorie consumption and still enjoy tasty, filling meals by putting these tips into practice. Try a variety of ingredients and cooking methods to see what suits your lifestyle and taste buds the best.

Chapter 6
Smart Snacks and Desserts

Guilt-Free Snack Ideas to Tame Your Cravings

Savor some fresh fruit, such as grapes, berries, oranges, bananas, or apples. Fruits are normally sweet and a great source of fiber, vitamins, and minerals.

Vegetables Sticks and Humus: For a filling, high-fiber, high-protein snack, dunk sliced carrots, cucumbers, bell peppers, or celeriac sticks into creamy hummus.

Greek Yogurt with Berries: For a creamy and wholesome snack rich in protein and antioxidants, combine Greek yogurt with your preferred berries, including strawberries, blueberries, or raspberries.

Combined Nuts and Seeds: To make your own trail mix, mix together several kinds of nuts and seeds, including sunflower, cashew, walnut, and almond. Nuts and seeds have high in fiber, protein, and good fats.

Whole Grains Crackers with Avocado: For a filling snack high in fiber and healthy fats, spread mashed avocado over crackers made with whole grains and season with a little salt and black pepper.

Popcorn: A crispy, low-calorie snack choice is air-popped popcorn. Savor it unseasoned or add flavor with a dash of dietary yeast, cinnamon, or other preferred spices.

Hard-Boiled Eggs: An easy and high-protein snack choice is hard-boiled eggs. Savor them as is on their own, or add a dash of pepper and sea salt for a little more taste.

Edamame: Edamame, or young soybeans, are a delightful, high-protein snack that is also high in fibre and antioxidant. Simply steam or boil the soybeans and season with little sea salt before serving.

Rice Cake and Peanut Butter: For a filling snack that blends creamy nut butters with crunchy whole grains, spread natural peanut oil or almond butter atop a rice cake.

Freeze grapes to enjoy a naturally sweet and refreshing snack. Use them to make ice chunks in your preferred beverage or just eat them straight out of the freezer.

These healthy, tasty, and filling guilt-free snack options are ideal for sating cravings in between meals. Always pay attention to your body's signals of hunger and fullness and select foods that are going to please your taste buds and fuel your body

Low-Calorie Dessert Recipes for Sweet Tooth Satisfaction

This easy dessert dish is minimal in calories and can fulfill your sweet desire without breaking the bank:

Bits of frozen bananas

Ingredients

a. Two fully ripe bananas

b. One-fourth cup of dark chocolate chips

c. One tablespoon of coconut oil

d. Sprinkles, crushed coconut, and chopped almonds are optional garnishes.

Instructions

After peeling, chop the bananas into small pieces.

The banana chunks should be frozen for approximately an hour, or until firm, on a baking sheet covered with parchment paper.

Put the coconut oil and dark chocolate chips in a dish that is safe to microwave. Microwave the chocolate for 30 seconds at a time, stirring throughout, until it melts and becomes smooth.

Take your frozen banana pieces out of the freezer, and then dip them all into the chocolaty mixture, being sure to completely cover each bite of banana with a fork.

Reposition the chocolate-covered banana bits on the baking sheet covered with parchment paper.

You may top the banana bits using chopped nuts, chopped coconut, or sprinkles, if you'd like.

Put the baking sheet back in the freezer and let it stay there for a further one to two hours, to ensure the chocolate sets.

The frozen banana bits may be kept in the fridge until they're time to serve by transferring them to an air tight container once the chocolate has solidified.

Enjoy these bite-sized frozen bananas as a guilt-free snack or dessert every time you're in the mood for something sweet! They're a flavorful, low-calorie treat that's still filling and delightful.

Mindful Eating Techniques for Enjoying Snacks in Moderation

Stop and Evaluate Your Hunger: Consider your degree of hunger for a moment prior to reaching for a snack. Consider whether you're eating because of habit, boredom, or stress rather than whether you're actually hungry.

Select Nutrient-Dense Foods

Choose foods that will fill you up and satiate your appetite instead of ones that are just empty calories. Pick foods high in nutrients, such as whole grain crackers, nuts, seeds, fruits, and vegetables.

Control of Portion

When you nibble, pay attention to the portion amounts. Measure out a portion of food into a dish or plate as opposed to aimlessly eating from a huge bag or container. This enables you to delight in your snack in moderation and helps prevent overeating.

Eat Without Distractions: Steer clear of snacking when preoccupied with work, devices, or other activities. Rather, schedule a certain time for snacking, when you can ignore all other distractions and concentrate just on enjoying your meal.

Involve Your Senses

While enjoying your food, spend the time to use all of your senses. Take note of the food's tastes, textures, colors, and aromas. Take note of the flavors and textures that each mouthful brings to your tongue.

Chew gently and mindfully

Savor the tastes and textures of every single chew of your snack by chewing it gently and deliberately. Eating slowly helps you avoid overeating by allowing your body to recognize emotions of contentment and fullness.

Pay Attention to Your Body

When you snack, pay attention to your body's signals of hunger and fullness. Rather than eating until the meal is gone or out of habit, stop eating when you're pleasantly full.

Exercise Gratitude

Give yourself a moment to be thankful for the delicious snack and the nutrition it contains. Developing an attitude of thankfulness can improve your connection with food and increase your pleasure of it.

Conscious Breathing

Before and after having your snack, take a few slow breaths to help you relax yourself and bring your attention to the here and now. In addition to lowering stress, mindful breathing may foster contentment and tranquility.

Consider Your Satisfaction

Once you've consumed your snack, pause to consider your feelings. Take note of any lingering hunger or emotions of contentment or pleasure. Make use of this knowledge to inform your future dietary decisions.

You may enjoy your favorite goodies in moderation and foster a better connection with food and eating by implementing these mindful eating practices into your snack routine.

Conclusion

Taking Stock of Your Calorie Deficit Experience

A crucial step in the process is to reflect on the calorie reduction trip. This will enable you to evaluate your progress, draw lessons from your mistakes, and make any improvements. Here's a way to think back on your experience with calorie deficit:

Celebrate Your Accomplishments: Regardless of how minor your accomplishments may seem, take a minute to recognize and honor them. Acknowledging your success may help you feel more motivated and self-assured, whether it's about reaching a weight reduction goal, adopting a healthier lifestyle, or getting fitter.

Assess Difficulties: Consider the difficulties you have faced when following a calorie deficit. Think back to the challenges you overcame, including hunger pangs, emotional eating, or peer pressure. Recognizing obstacles enables you to create plans for conquering them later on.

Evaluate Compliance: Examine how well you've followed your calorie-deficit strategy. Did you maintain a regular food diary and adhere to your calorie target? Did you ever find it difficult to follow through on your plan? You may find areas for improvement and, if necessary, change your approach by evaluating your compliance.

Track Your Progress: Whether your objective is to lose weight, improve your body composition, or improve your general health, track your progress toward it. To precisely monitor your progress, think about utilizing objective metrics like evaluations, body fat percentages, or results from physical activities.

Consider Non-Scale successes: Consider the non-scale successes you have had by looking past the scale's numbers. This might entail enhancements in mood, energy levels, confidence, quality of sleep, or general wellbeing. Non-scale successes can serve as a useful source of inspiration to carry on with your journey, since they are frequently just as significant as weight changes.

Learn from obstacles: Consider any mistakes or obstacles you've encountered on your journey. Consider them as chances for learning and development rather than as failures. Determine what caused the setback and come up with ideas for better ways to handle such circumstances in the future.

Reevaluate Your Objectives: Give your objectives a second look in the context of your observations. Do your objectives still seem doable and reasonable? Do you desire to change your strategy or your timeframe in any way? You may maintain your motivation and attention while pursuing your weight-loss journey by reevaluating your objectives.

Exercise Self-Compassion: Treat yourself with kindness while you contemplate. Keep in mind that it takes patience, effort, and time to bring about long-lasting change. Rather of being unduly judgmental of yourself, learn to be compassionate with yourself and accept that obstacles are a normal part of the process.

Seek Support: For accountability and encouragement, reach out to relatives, close companions, or a supportive community. Talking to others about your observations might yield insightful comments as well as keep you motivated and goal-focused.

Adapt and Adjust: Modify your calorie deficit strategy as needed in light of your thoughts. This might entail changing your diet, getting more exercise, or getting help from a licensed dietitian or other healthcare provider. Never forget that long-term success depends on your capacity to adjust and be flexible.

You may obtain important insights, maintain motivation, and make wise decisions that will ultimately promote your general well-being and health by routinely meditating on your low-calorie journey.

Celebrating Your Achievements and Progress

Celebrating your victories and advancements is a crucial component of continuing to be inspired and to keep moving forward on your path. Here are some heartfelt ideas for commemorating your accomplishments:

Establish Milestones: Divide your more ambitious objectives into more doable, smaller benchmarks. Whether it's reaching a weight loss goal, finishing a fitness difficulty, or adhering to the calorie-reduction plan for a predetermined amount of time, celebrate each accomplishment as a milestone.

Reward Yourself: After reaching a goal, treat yourself to something special. Select incentives that fit your beliefs and aspirations, such purchasing new exercise equipment, scheduling a spa day, or treating yourself to a special dinner at your preferred restaurant (while still keeping an eye on your calorie deficit targets).

Record Your Development: Maintain a visual record of your accomplishments and advancement. Make a progress notebook where you may note your achievements, track modifications to your level of fitness, and record measurements. Observing your progress may be immensely inspiring.

Share Your Success: Let your family, friends, or a caring community know what you've accomplished. Celebrate your accomplishments with those closest to you, who can encourage you and feel your excitement. In order to encourage other people on their own travels, you may also share your achievement on social networks or in online forums.

Create a Fitness Challenge for Yourself: Take on a new exercise regimen or set a new fitness objective.

Reaching a fitness goal may be a satisfying way to recognize your advancement, whether it's finishing a 5K race, learning a new yoga posture, or lifting more weight at the gym.

Make a Vision Board: Using a vision board can help you visualize your objectives and dreams. Add pictures, sayings, and affirmations that uplift you and symbolize your accomplishments. Put your vision board somewhere noticeable so you can view it every day and be reminded of your goals.

Honor Non-Scale Victories: Honor accomplishments that surpass the scale's numerical values. Acknowledge gains in your general well-being, energy, mood, and confidence. These successes outside of the scale are equally significant as weight loss and should be honored.

Practice Gratitude: Give yourself a time to be thankful for all of your accomplishments and the strides you've achieved. Think back on the improvements you've seen and the knowledge you've picked up along the road. Developing an attitude of thankfulness can make the journey more enjoyable for you and motivate you to keep going.

Pay It Forward: Show your gratitude for your accomplishments by showing compassion and charity to others. Contribute voluntarily, make a charity donation, or provide assistance and motivation to others pursuing their own goals. Talking about your accomplishments with others might make you feel even more happy about it and spread optimism throughout the community.

Recall that honoring your efforts and commitment to your path is just as important as accomplishing your goals when it comes to celebrating your accomplishments. Recognize and appreciate your accomplishments, since each one will move you one step closer to your final goals

Tips for Maintaining Weight Loss and Healthy Habits Long-Term

Long-term weight loss and the maintenance of good behaviors need commitment, regularity, and a sustainable strategy. The following intriguing advice can assist you in continuing to make improvement over time:

Prioritize Sustainable improvements: Rather than focusing on fad diets or fast solutions, prioritize implementing sustainable lifestyle improvements. Make healthy food choices you appreciate, engage in physical activity you enjoy, and create long-lasting habits.

Eat with awareness: During meals, pay close attention to what your body is saying signals of hunger and fullness. Eat mindfully, enjoy every meal, and halt when you're full, not full-blown. A better relationship with food and the avoidance of overeating are two benefits of mindful eating.

Remain Active: To support the maintenance of your weight reduction and general health, include regular physical exercise in your daily routine. Whether it be walking, cycling, to swim, or dancing, find something you want to do and try to get in at least 150 minutes a week of moderate-intensity activity.

Establish Achievable, Realistic Goals: Make sure your objectives suit your talents, preferences, and way of life. Divide more ambitious objectives into more doable steps, and acknowledge each accomplishment as it occurs.

Realistic goal-setting keeps motivation high and helps shield against burnout

Seek Assistance: Assemble a network of friends, family, or other health-conscious individuals who will support and inspire you along the way. Other helpful resources for accountability and support include working with a wellness coach, joining a support community, and taking part in online communities.

Track Your Progress: Keep an eye on your weight, measurements, degree of fitness, and other pertinent indicators to be informed about your progress. Continually evaluate your performance and make necessary habit adjustments to stay on course. Monitoring your development enables you to spot patterns, recognize accomplishments, and pinpoint areas in need of development.

Plan Ahead: To assist you in making better decisions throughout the day, schedule food and snacks in advance. Ensure your kitchen is stocked with wholesome ingredients, cook in large quantities, and carry wholesome snacks for on-the-go. Making a plan lowers the chance of impulsive snacking and guarantees that you have wholesome alternatives on hand.

Practice Self-Care: Make self-care activities a priority in order to look after your mental, emotional, and physical health. Make time for enjoyable hobbies, get enough sleep, and use relaxation methods like deep breathing or meditation to handle stress. Long-term maintenance of a healthy lifestyle is facilitated by comprehensive self-care.

Celebrate Non-Scale Victories: Take note of and give thanks for any non-scale successes you may have encountered along the way, such as more confidence, higher energy, happier moods, or better sleep. These are accomplishments that should be honored and appreciated, just as significant as weight loss.

Be Compassionate to Yourself: Show yourself kindness and self-compassion, even when things are hard. Recall that mistakes are acceptable and that obstacles are a normal part of the path. Focus on development rather than perfection, and treat yourselves with the same consideration and compassion that you would show a friend.

You may sustain your weight reduction and good behaviors over time by putting these amazing recommendations into practice, which will enhance your general well-being and health for generations to come.